THE ULTIMATE MEN'S HEALTH GUIDE

Your Roadmap to a Healthier, Happier Life

C. ANGLIN

Table of Contents

CHAPTER 1
INTRODUCTION TO MEN'S HEALTH

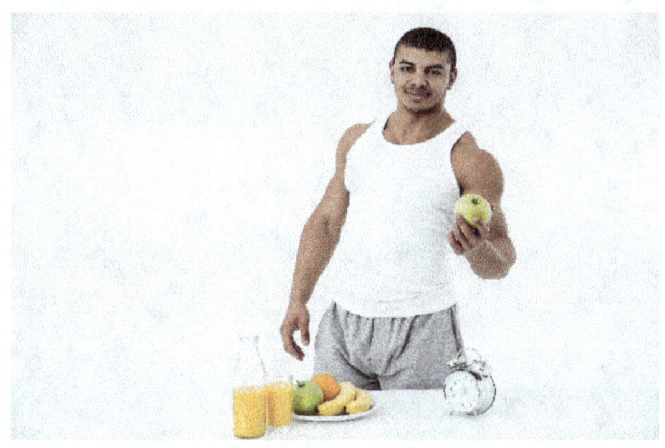

Optimal health is a critical aspect of overall well-being. It is essential to maintain a healthy lifestyle to prevent various health issues. In this chapter, we will discuss the importance of men's health and why it is crucial to prioritize it. We will also provide an overview of the book's contents and how it can help men maintain good health. Maintaining good health is essential for men of all ages. It is crucial to prioritize your health and well-being to prevent various health issues. In this chapter, we will discuss the importance of men's health and why it is crucial to prioritize it. We will also provide an overview of the book's contents and how it can help men maintain good health.

It is important for men to prioritize health because it is vital to their overall well-being, performance, and quality of life. Good health enables men to carry out daily activities, enjoy life to the fullest, and sustain a positive lifestyle. Examples of prioritizing health include eating a balanced diet, exercising regularly, getting adequate sleep, and scheduling regular health check-ups. Additionally, men should pay special attention to their mental and emotional health too, by engaging in activities such as therapy, mindfulness, and meditation. Taking good care of one's health has long-lasting benefits, such as reduced risk of chronic diseases, increased energy levels, and improved mood and self-esteem.

CHAPTER 2
NUTRITION AND DIET

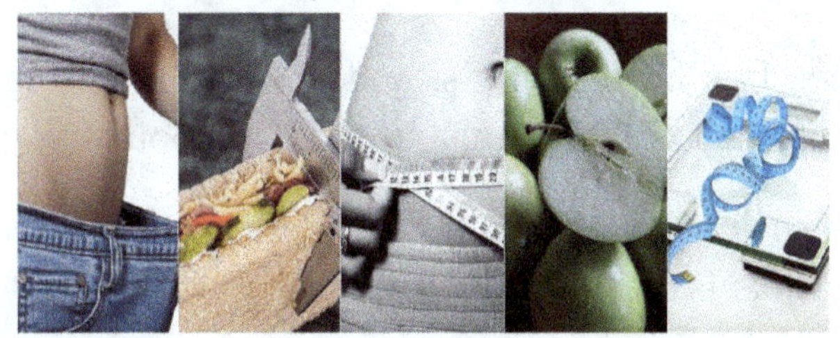

Maintaining a healthy diet is essential for men of all ages. In this chapter, we will discuss the importance of a balanced diet and provide tips on how to make healthy food choices. We will also provide an in-depth look at the different food groups and how they contribute to overall health. Additionally, we will discuss the importance of portion control and how to maintain a healthy weight. We will also provide a list of healthy recipes and meal plans to help men maintain a healthy diet.

To maintain optimal health and combat the risk of certain health conditions. Here are some healthy food choices to help optimize men's health:

- Get your greens and other veggies; along with fruit, whole grains, lean meats, nuts, and dairy or dairy alternatives - these will help supercharge your diet.

- Fruits are a great source of vitamins, fiber, and antioxidants that can help reduce the risk of chronic diseases.

- Select unrefined whole-grain bread and cereals instead of those containing refined flour. Whole grains are a top choice for healthy prostate and muscle health.

- Lean meats such as chicken, turkey, and fish are excellent protein sources that can help build and maintain muscle mass.

- Almonds, walnuts, pecans, cashews, pistachios, and peanuts have healthy fats, protein, and fiber that you'd like to give a try.

- Enjoy fish like salmon, rainbow trout, and Atlantic mackerel, limited in mercury and rich with omega-3 fats, which can help lower the risk of diabetes and heart disease.

- Legumes like beans, lentils, and chickpeas are high in nutrients including fiber and protein, a healthy addition to your diet.

- Berries such as blueberries, strawberries, and raspberries are high in antioxidants and can help lower inflammation in your body.

- Savor the taste of bananas, they're an excellent source of potassium that naturally lowers blood pressure and reduces the risk of heart disease.

- Don't forget dairy products like milk, cheese, and yogurt. They are great sources of calcium, which is crucial in keeping your bones healthy.

Remember to reduce the intake of foods high in saturated fats, added salts & sugars, and alcohol for a healthy diet.

Recipes and meal plan ideas:

Breakfast:

Idli (steamed lentil cakes) with Coconut Chutney.

Scrambled Egg Omelets with Spinach, Tomatoes, and Garlic – 2 eggs, 3 tablespoons of spinach, and fresh chopped tomatoes

Lunch:

Quinoa and Black Bean Salad – 1 cup quinoa, 1/4 cup black beans

Grilled Chicken Breast with Roasted Asparagus – 4oz of chicken breast, 8 spears of asparagus

Snack:

Apple with Almond Butter – 1 large apple, 2 tablespoons of almond butter

Dinner:

Baked Salmon Filet – 4oz Salmon filet

Steamed Broccoli with Olive Oil – 4 cups of broccoli, 1 tablespoon of olive oil.

Meal Plan:

Monday:

Breakfast: Idli (steamed lentil cakes) with Coconut Chutney

Lunch: Quinoa and Black Bean Salad

Snack: Apple with Almond Butter

Dinner: Baked Salmon Filet with Steamed Broccoli

Tuesday:

Breakfast: Scrambled Egg Omelets with Spinach, Tomatoes, and Garlic

Lunch: Grilled Chicken Breast with Roasted Asparagus

Snack: Hummus and Celery Sticks - 2 tablespoons of hummus, 4 stalks of celery

Dinner: Shrimp and Vegetable Stir Fry – 6oz shrimp, 2 cups of stir-fried vegetables

Wednesday:

Breakfast: Overnight Oats with Mixed Berries – 1/2 cup of old-fashioned oats, 1/4 cup of mixed berries

Lunch: Lentil Soup – 1 cup of lentil soup

Snack: Greek Yogurt with Nut Granola – 2/3 cup of Greek yogurt, 2 tablespoons of nut granola

Dinner: Grilled Vegetable and Quinoa Bowl – 1 cup of quinoa, a mix of 2 cups diced vegetables.

Thursday:

Breakfast: Toast with Avocado and Tomatoes – 2 slices of whole-wheat toast, 1 avocado, and slices of fresh tomatoes

Lunch: Chickpea and Spinach Salad – 1/2 cup of chickpeas, 2 cups of baby spinach

Snack: Apple slices with Peanut Butter – 2 slices of apple, 1 tablespoon of peanut butter

Dinner: Roasted Turkey with Brussels Sprouts – 4oz of roasted turkey, 8 Brussels sprouts

Friday:

Breakfast: Scrambled Egg Whites with Mushrooms – 2 egg whites, 4 chopped mushrooms

Lunch: Kale and Brown Rice Bowl – 1 cup of brown rice, 1 cup of kale

Snack: Fruit Smoothie – 1 cup of frozen fruit, 1/2 cup of almond milk

Dinner: Baked Sweet Potatoes with Lentils – 1 large, sweet potato, 1/2 cup of cooked lentils

Saturday:

Breakfast: Banana Pancakes – 2 pancakes made with mashed banana and oats

Lunch: Salad with Tuna – 2 cups of lettuce or mixed greens, 4oz of canned tuna

Snack: Carrots with Hummus – 4 carrots, 2 tablespoons of hummus

Dinner: Vegetable Curry – 2 cups of diced vegetables in curry sauce

Sunday:

Breakfast: Whole Grain Toast with Peanut Butter and Banana – 2 slices of whole grain toast, 1 tablespoon of peanut butter, 1 banana

Lunch: Tomato and Mozzarella Sandwich – 2 slices of whole grain bread, 1/2 cup of sliced tomatoes, 3 slices of mozzarella cheese

Snack: Celery with Cream Cheese – 4 crystals of celery, 2 tablespoons of cream cheese

Dinner: Grilled Vegetables and Quinoa Bowl – 1 cup of quinoa, 2 cups of diced vegetables

Helpful Websites:

- ChooseMyPlate.gov
- EatRight.org
- Nutrition.gov

CHAPTER 3
EXERCISE AND FITNESS

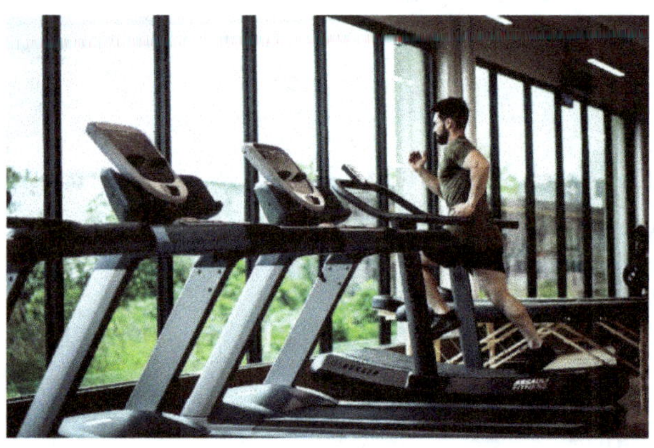

Regular exercise is crucial for maintaining good health. Are you ready to learn about the benefits of exercise and how to incorporate physical activity into your daily routine? This chapter not only provides the different types of exercises that are beneficial for men's health but also highlights the importance of stretching and injury prevention during exercise. To ensure that you can stay on track and maintain a healthy exercise routine, we have included a list of recommended exercises and workout plans. Let's get started on the path to a healthier you!

Discovering new ways to stay fit and healthy can be a fun challenge, and luckily, there are countless exercises and fitness activities that you can do from the comfort of your own home, even without any specialized equipment. Whether you're a fan of gentle stretching or prefer high-intensity workouts, there's something for everyone. Try jogging in place, sitting in a squat or pike position, or even dancing to your favorite tunes. If you're looking for a more social experience, consider joining a group fitness class or trying out an online class. You can even incorporate physical activity into your daily routine by doing tasks like cleaning, gardening, or walking. By embracing these different fitness options, you'll not only feel better physically but also mentally, as you're engaging in activities that promote overall wellness.

Aerobic exercises are beneficial for overall health. Examples include running, cycling, swimming, walking, and dancing. Other types of exercise that can be beneficial are strength training, yoga, and Pilates. To begin any of these exercise routines, it is important to consult with a healthcare professional to ensure that it is the most suitable type of exercise for your body. Once you have your doctor's approval, the following steps are recommended:

1. Start with warm-up exercises such as stretching and jogging in place.

2. Begin with low-impact, safe exercises, and gradually work your way up to more challenging activities.

3. Pay attention to form and focus on breathing with each exercise to help reduce the risk of injury.

4. Make sure to rest at least 1-2 days per week.

5. Drink plenty of water and refuel with a healthy snack before and after workouts.

6. Get enough sleep to allow the body to recover after exercise.

Examples of strength training for men

Strength training is beneficial for men as it helps build muscle, strengthen bones, reduce body fat, and improve overall fitness. Examples of strength training exercises for men include:

1. Push-ups

2. Pull-ups

3. Squats

4. Lunges

5. Crunches

6. Bullworker

7. Weightlifting

8. Plyometrics

9. High-intensity interval training (HIIT)

Helpful Websites:

- CDC.gov/PhysicalActivity

- ACEfitness.org

- Bodybuilding.com

CHAPTER 4
MENTAL HEALTH

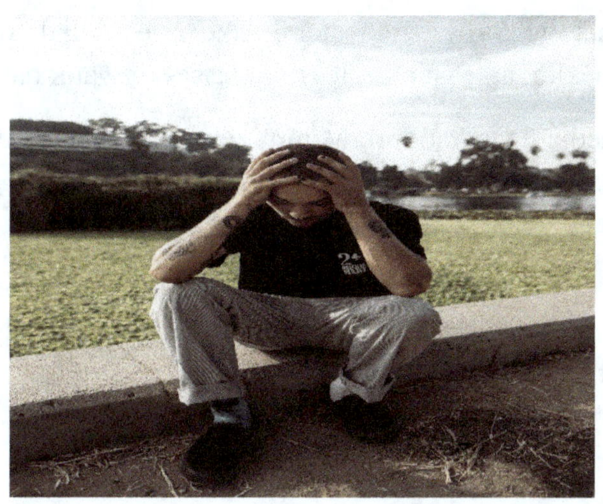

Taking care of your mental health is just as crucial as keeping your body fit and strong. Dive into this captivating chapter where we unveil the significance of mental well-being while offering handy tips to stay mentally fit. Unravel an extensive analysis of various mental health challenges men encounter, such as depression and anxiety. Moreover, emphasize the value of reaching out to professionals when required. Maintaining sound mental health is vital for men throughout their lives, and this chapter is packed with essential guidance for those who may be grappling with mental health concerns. You will also discover a treasure trove of resources tailored specifically for men in need.

Here are some daily habits that can greatly enhance men's mental health, accompanied by illustrative examples:

Prioritize sleep: Acquiring a good night's sleep is crucial for mental well-being. Strive for 7-8 hours of restorative sleep each evening.

Stay active: Engaging in regular physical activity can do wonders for your mental health. Intense workouts aren't a must; even seated exercises, hourly stretching, gardening, or leisurely walks contribute to mental wellness.

Eat nutritiously: A well-balanced diet plays a significant role in promoting mental health. Opt for wholesome meals like yogurt with nuts and berries, vegetable omelets, or low-sugar granola bars paired with fresh fruit.

Hydrate adequately. Sufficient water intake is essential for maintaining sound mental health. at least or at least 8 glasses of water daily.

Limit social media consumption: Minimizing social media usage can help alleviate its detrimental effects on mental health. Take breaks whenever possible and set boundaries around time spent online.

Cultivate mindfulness: Embracing mindfulness techniques assists in stress reduction and mental health improvement. Experiment with meditation, deep breathing exercises, or yoga to discover your preferred mindfulness method.

Foster connections: Social relationships are vital for positive mental health. Reach out to friends and family, participate in clubs or groups, or volunteer in your local community to stay connected.

Take regular breaks: Periodic rest breaks throughout the day help alleviate stress and bolster mental well-being. Brief walks stretch, or deep-breathing practices make for excellent pauses.

Organize your day: Daily planning promotes stress reduction and enhances productivity. Create to-do lists or utilize planners to keep yourself organized and on track.

Prioritize self-care: Self-care plays a crucial role in fostering good mental health. Enjoy some peaceful moments by taking a warm bath, reading an engaging book, or indulging in a cherished hobby.

Embrace nature: Immersing yourself in the great outdoors can alleviate stress and bolster mental health. Explore your surroundings by walking, hiking, or camping to soak up nature's therapeutic benefits.

Absorb sunlight: Sunlight exposure significantly influences mental health. Endeavor to spend time outdoors each day or, in areas with limited sunshine, consider a light therapy box to emulate natural light.

Helpful Websites:

- NAMI.org

- MentalHealth.gov

- PsychologyToday.com

CHAPTER 5
SEXUAL HEALTH

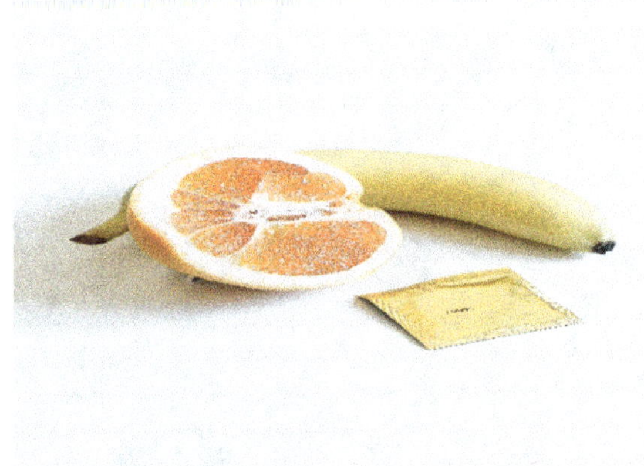

Good sexual health is essential for men of all ages. In this chapter, we will discuss the importance of sexual health and provide tips on how to maintain good sexual health. We will also provide an in-depth look at different sexual health issues that men may face, such as erectile dysfunction and premature ejaculation. Additionally, we will discuss the importance of safe sex practices and how to prevent sexually transmitted infections. We will also provide a list of resources for men who may be struggling with sexual health issues.

Boost your sexual prowess with these daily habits and tips designed to optimize men's sexual health based on expert advice:

1. Make foreplay a priority: Many men assume that penetration is the key to great sex; however, indulging in sensual foreplay can

heighten the pleasure and satisfaction of both partners.

2. Master the start-stop technique: By momentarily halting sexual activity just before orgasm and resuming after a short pause, you can enhance control and prolong ejaculation.

3. Keep anxiety and stress at bay: As these factors can impair sexual performance, practice stress-management techniques like exercising, meditation, or engaging in relaxing hobbies to maintain a robust sex life.

4. Commit to consistent exercise: A regular fitness regimen not only improves overall health but also bolsters stamina for stellar sexual encounters. Plus, exercise contributes to better mental health and reduced anxiety.

5. Perform Kegel workouts: These exercises target the pelvic floor muscles, strengthening bladder control and promoting healthy sexual function.

6. Savor a nutritious diet: Consuming antioxidant-rich foods like fruits and vegetables as well as omega-3 fatty acid sources such as fish supports both general health and sexual vitality.

7. Prioritize proper sleep: Adequate rest benefits overall wellness and enhances sexual function by combating fatigue and low libido.

8. Limit alcohol and drug consumption: Minimizing or abstaining from these substances can dramatically improve your sexual prowess, as they often impair your performance.

9. Consult a medical professional: Should you face persistent sexual challenges, open communication with your doctor can help uncover any underlying issues and appropriate treatment strategies.

Studies have found that regular sex can have a significant positive impact on men's physical and mental health. Sex helps to release endorphins, which are hormones that increase the feeling of happiness and well-being. This can help to reduce stress levels and improve overall emotional health. Sex also helps to strengthen the immune system, helping men to fight off illnesses and stay healthy. Furthermore, it contributes to muscle relaxation and improved circulation, helping to lower blood pressure and reduce the risk of heart disease. Regular sex can also help men to maintain strong erectile function, promoting sexual health.

Incorporating these effective routines and recommendations will not only optimize your sexual health but also elevate your overall quality of life.

Helpful Websites:

- CDC.gov/STD

- PlannedParenthood.org

- SexualHealth.com

CHAPTER 6
SLEEP

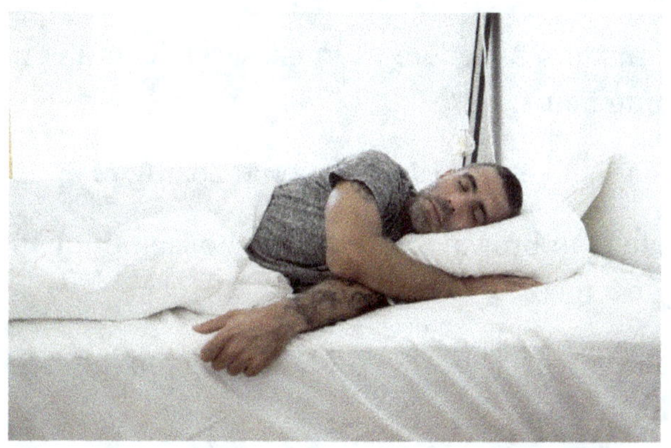

Securing a good night's sleep is paramount for upholding optimal health. In this fascinating chapter, we will dive into the significance of sleep and furnish you with valuable tips to enhance your sleep quality. We will also embark on a comprehensive exploration of various sleep disorders that affect men, such as sleep apnea and insomnia, shedding light on their intricacies. Furthermore, we will emphasize the importance of establishing a robust sleep routine as a key component of healthy living. Mastering proper sleep habits is indispensable for men across all age groups. Not only will we delve into the crucial aspects of sleep and share practical advice for improving sleep quality, but we will additionally provide an extensive list of resources tailored to assist men who may be grappling with elusive slumber.

Boost your sleep game for a healthier life, guys! Check out these trending tips:

1. Be a creature of habit: Stick to a regular bedtime and wake-up schedule, even on weekends.

2. Create a snooze sanctuary: Keep your bedroom cool, dark, and quiet, and ditch those tech gadgets before bed.

3. Sidestep stimulants: Steer clear of caffeine, alcohol, and hefty meals before hitting the sack.

4. Get moving: Engage in daily physical activity to help make falling asleep at night a breeze.

5. Timing matters Schedule exercise sessions in the morning instead of evening hours.

6. Power nap like a pro: Limit daytime dozing to 20 minutes or less.

7. Moderate your brews: Keep alcohol consumption to under 2 drinks per day for men.

8. Ditch late-night feasts: Avoid loading up on food right before bedtime.

9. Unwind your mind: Jot down worries and to-do lists before bed to clear your head for sleep.

10. Establish a bedtime ritual: A consistent sleep schedule and relaxing routine help regulate your body's sleep cycle for easy sleeping and waking.

By embracing these suggestions, men can enhance their sleep quality, leading to improved overall health and well-being!

Common sleep disorders include insomnia, sleep apnea, and restless leg syndrome. Treatment for sleep disorders may include therapy, medication, and lifestyle changes such as maintaining a consistent sleep schedule and avoiding caffeine and alcohol before bedtime.

Helpful Websites:

- SleepFoundation.org

- American Academy of Sleep Medicine: https://aasm.org/

- NationalSleepFoundation.org

- SleepEducation.org

CHAPTER 7
HEART HEALTH

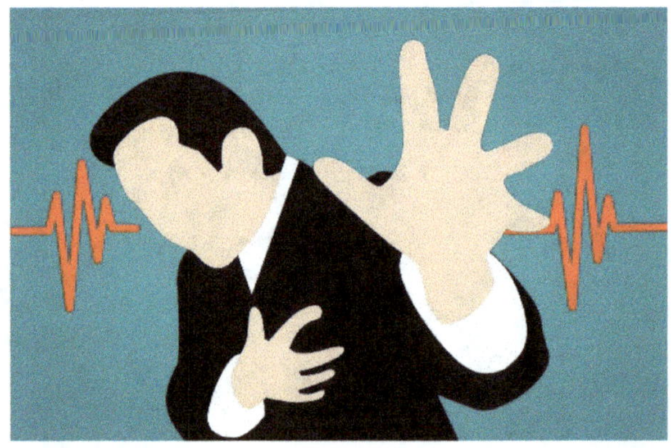

Cardiovascular disease is a predominant cause of mortality among the male population. In this section, we shall delve into the significance of maintaining optimal cardiovascular well-being and offer guidance on how to promote good heart health. Furthermore, we will furnish an exhaustive analysis of various cardiac conditions that men may encounter, such as elevated blood pressure and coronary artery disease. Additionally, the necessity of consistent medical examinations and screenings will be emphasized. We will also supply an array of resources for individuals who may be grappling with heart-related ailments. Optimizing men's heart health is crucial in today's fast-paced world. Let's dive into the top measures every man should take to boost heart health and embrace a fulfilling lifestyle:

1. Embrace a heart-healthy diet: Choosing fiber-rich whole grains, vibrant fruits, and vegetables, and incorporating healthy fats from sources like olive oil significantly enhances heart health.

2. Maintain an ideal weight: Staying within a healthy weight range reduces the chances of heart disease. Striking a balance between nutritious eating habits and regular exercise is the key.

3. Incorporate daily physical activities: Aiming for 30-60 minutes of daily exercise, such as brisk walking, biking, or swimming, boosts not only cardiovascular health but also overall well-being.

4. Say no to smoking and tobacco: These habits significantly raise the risk of heart condition. Quitting tobacco use and avoiding secondhand smoke are non-negotiable steps toward better heart health.

5. Regulate cholesterol and blood pressure levels: Elevated cholesterol and blood pressure can be detrimental to one's heart. Eating right, staying active, and using medications (if required) effectively manage these levels.

6. Curb sodium consumption: To prevent hypertension and safeguard your heart, consciously reduce daily sodium intake.

7. Tackle stress head-on: Stress can silently fuel heart complications. Confront stress with regular exercise, relaxation techniques such as deep breathing or meditation, and relying on your support network of friends and family.

By consistently practicing these measures, men can significantly improve their heart health while minimizing the risk of cardiovascular diseases. Embrace this trending approach toward a healthier, more fulfilling life!

Helpful Websites:

- Heart.org

- CDC.gov/HeartDisease

- MayoClinic.org/Heart-Disease

CHAPTER 8
ADDRESSING STRESS

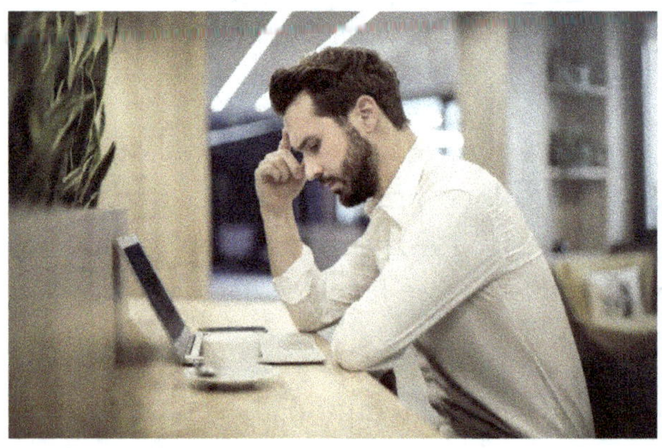

It is critically important for men to reduce stress in their lives because excessive and prolonged stress can be harmful in various ways. Stress increases the production of stress hormones, such as cortisol and adrenaline, which can cause physical health problems such as high blood pressure, digestive problems, headaches, depression, and difficulty sleeping. High levels of stress can also take an emotional toll with fatigue, irrational anger, guilt, anxiety, and more. In the long term, chronic stress can often result in serious medical conditions such as heart disease, stroke, diabetes, and some mental health conditions.

Reducing stress can provide overall health benefits and improve quality of life. Practicing stress relief techniques can help men develop the skills to better manage stress and their reactions to it. Mindfulness meditation, yoga, and tai chi are all excellent ways to learn how to remain calm and centered in the face of challenging situations and emotions. Deep breathing exercises and progressive muscle relaxation can both help to reduce the physical effects of stress like a rapid heart rate or tense muscles. Physical exercise is an excellent way to reduce stress as it boosts endorphins and can work to clear your head. Other activities such as engaging in hobbies, nurturing meaningful relationships, and enjoying pleasant activities like listening to music can also be helpful.

Resources to learn more about stress relief can often be found in your local community or online. Self-help books, websites, podcasts, and counseling are all good options. The important thing is to take the time to create an individualized plan to make sure that stress is managed in a healthy way. Taking the time to practice stress-reducing activities can ultimately reduce health risks and help lead to improved physical and mental well-being.

In a study conducted by the CDC in 2019, it was estimated that the prevalence of stress is much higher in men than in women across the United States. Approximately 25% of men reported having frequent feelings of extreme stress in comparison to 19% of women. This indicates that men are more likely to suffer from the harmful effects of elevated stress, which can include both physical and psychological issues. When left untreated, this stress can have long-term consequences for a person's quality of life.

Stress can lead to physical health issues such as high blood pressure, heart disease, headaches, insomnia, and digestive problems. Additionally, it can result in poor mental health outcomes such as depression, anxiety, and irrational anger. Furthermore, research has shown that high levels of stress can increase the risk of addiction, suicidal behaviors, and even some chronic illnesses such as heart disease and stroke. Therefore, it is essential that men recognize and address the signs and symptoms of stress to reduce its potentially harmful effects and improve their overall well-being.

One way to reduce stress is to practice stress relief activities. Mindfulness meditation, yoga, and tai chi are all excellent methods for learning how to remain calm and centered during difficult situations. Deep breathing exercises and progressive muscle relaxation can also help reduce the physical effects of stress such as a rapid heart rate or tense muscles. Moreover, physical exercise is a great way to relieve stress as it can help boost endorphins and clear the head. Other activities such as engaging in hobbies, nurturing meaningful relationships, and enjoying pleasant activities like listening to music can be used to reduce stress levels as well.

Overall, it is necessary for men to be aware of and address the signs and symptoms of stress to reduce its potential harm and improve their well-being. Taking the time to develop an individualized and tailored plan to reduce stress is important so that men can reduce their health risks and enjoy the physical and mental benefits of a more balanced and fulfilled life.

CHAPTER 9
CANCER SUPPORT, RESOURCES, AND PREVENTION

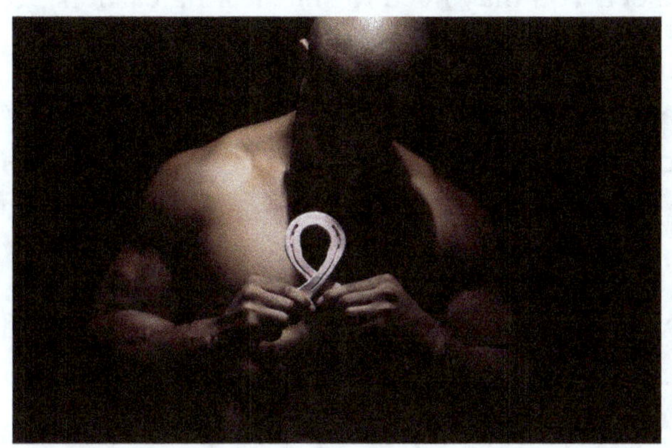

Cancer is a significant health concern for men and finding support during and after cancer treatment is essential for men of all ages. In this chapter, we will discuss the importance of cancer support and resources and provide tips on how to find support during and after cancer treatment. We will also provide a brief look at different types of cancer that men may face, such as prostate cancer and lung cancer. Additionally, we will discuss the importance of regular check-ups and screenings. We will also provide a list of resources for men who may be struggling with cancer.

Cancer prevention in men offers several ways to help reduce the risk of getting cancer. The best way to start is by maintaining a healthy lifestyle, including eating a healthy diet, exercising regularly, and avoiding tobacco use. Maintain regular screenings, know your risk factors for cancer, and talk with your doctor about what is right for you. Men should ensure their healthcare provider knows if they have any concerns about being tested for or having prostate cancer.

There are several cancer screening tests recommended for men. Here are some of the specific tests recommended from the search results:

Prostate cancer: The most common screening tests for prostate cancer are the prostate-specific antigen (PSA) blood test and the digital rectal exam (DRE). Most men may want to get a PSA test, and possibly a DRE, starting at age 50. If you're Black, have or may have a faulty BRCA1 or BRCA2 gene, or other men (especially those younger than 65) in your family have had prostate cancer, you may need to start testing earlier.

Colorectal cancer: Men ages 45 to 75 should be screened for colorectal cancer. There are several screening tests available, including a stool-based fecal occult blood test (gFOBT) or fecal immunochemical test (FIT) every year, a flexible sigmoidoscopy every 5 years, a colonoscopy every 10 years, or a CT colonography every 5 years.

Lung cancer: Annual testing with low dose computed tomography (LDCT) is recommended between ages 55 and 80 if you have smoked the equivalent of a pack.

Maintain a healthy lifestyle: Many things can affect your chance of getting cancer, and making healthy choices is one of the most important things you can do to avoid getting cancer.

1. This includes eating a healthy diet, exercising regularly, and avoiding tobacco use.
2. Get regular screenings: Getting the screening tests that are right for you is important for the early detection and treatment of cancer. Know your risk factors: Understanding your risk factors for cancer can help you take steps to prevent it. Some of the most common cancers in men are prostate, colorectal, lung, and skin cancers.
3. Prostate cancer prevention: Prostate cancer is the most common cancer in American men, except for skin cancers. African American men and Caribbean men of African ancestry are more likely to

develop it. The Prostate Cancer Foundation provides information on prostate cancer prevention.

4. Cancer prevention resources: The Centers for Disease Control and Prevention (CDC) provides a feature on cancer and men, which includes information on cancer prevention and screening.

5. The National Cancer Institute (NCI) provides information on cancer causes and prevention, including research articles on cancer causes and prevention.

6. The American Cancer Society provides cancer facts for men, including information on common cancers in men and what you can do to help prevent them or find them early.

7. The World Health Organization (WHO) provides information on cancer prevention, including key risk factors to avoid.

It's important to talk to your doctor about which screening tests are right for you based on your age, personal and family health history, and other risk factors.

Regular self-checks can help you spot testicular cancer early. Here's a simple guide for testicular self-examination:

Pick the right time: Do the exam after a warm bath or shower when the scrotum is relaxed.

Stand before a mirror: Look for swelling or changes in the scrotum's skin. Check for lumps, bumps, or size and shape changes.

Check each testicle separately: Gently hold one testicle with thumbs and fingers. It's fine if one is bigger than the other.

Notice texture and shape: Softly roll the testicle between your fingers. Feel for hard lumps, irregularities, or size and shape changes. It should be smooth and firm, like a hard-boiled egg without its shell.

Find the epididymis: It's a soft, tube-like part behind the testicle. Don't mistake it for a lump or abnormality.

Examine the other testicle: Do the same process with the other one. Be thorough and check both individually.

Look out for pain or discomfort: Pay attention to any pain, discomfort, or heaviness during examination.

Do it every month: Regularly check your testicles, ideally monthly, to get familiar with their normal size, shape, and feel. This helps you notice any unusual changes.

Keep in mind that not all lumps or irregularities are cancerous – most are harmless. But if you find anything unusual during self-examination, see a healthcare professional for further evaluation and guidance.

Helpful Websites:

- Cancer.org
- CancerCare.org
- FloridaHealth.gov

CHAPTER 10
SUBSTANCE ABUSE AND ADDICTION

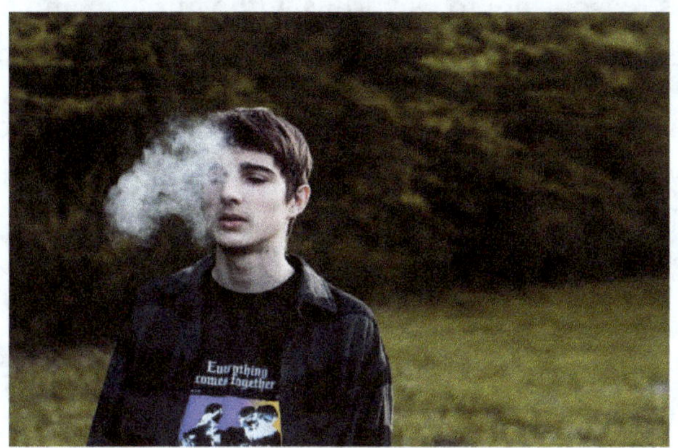

Addressing substance abuse and addiction is essential for men of all ages. We will discuss the importance of substance abuse and addiction prevention and provide tips on how to reduce your risk of addiction. We will also provide a brief look at different types of substance abuse and addiction that men may face, such as alcoholism and drug addiction. Additionally, we will discuss the importance of seeking professional help when needed. We will also provide a list of resources for men who may be struggling with substance abuse and addiction.

Substance abuse and addiction can have serious consequences for men. Here are some tips and strategies to prevent substance abuse and addiction:

Understand how substance abuse develops.

1. Avoid temptation and peer pressure by developing healthy friendships and relationships.

2. Seek help for mental illness.

3. Examine the risk factors that may lead to substance abuse, such as family history, trauma, and stress.

4. Keep a well-balanced life by practicing stress management skills and focusing on your goals and dreams for the future.

5. Mobilize the community and create awareness that addiction is a disease, that it is treatable, and that treatment is available.

6. Discuss reasons not to use drugs with your teen and emphasize how drug use can affect the things that are important to them.

7. Establish rules and consequences with your teen, such as leaving a party where drug use occurs and not riding in a car with a driver who's been using drugs.

8. Know your teen's activities and pay attention to their whereabouts.

9. Provide support and offer praise and encouragement when your teen succeeds.

10. Educate yourself and others about substance use disorder (SUD) and seek help as soon as you develop signs of SUD.

11. Utilize substance abuse prevention measures, such as planning, hoping, and dreaming about your future, and tracking your progress toward your goals.

12. Treat addicts and prevent the onset of drug use by expanding research in drug abuse prevention.

Helpful Websites:

- SAMHSA.gov

- DrugAbuse.gov

- AA.org

CHAPTER 11
MEN'S REPRODUCTIVE HEALTH

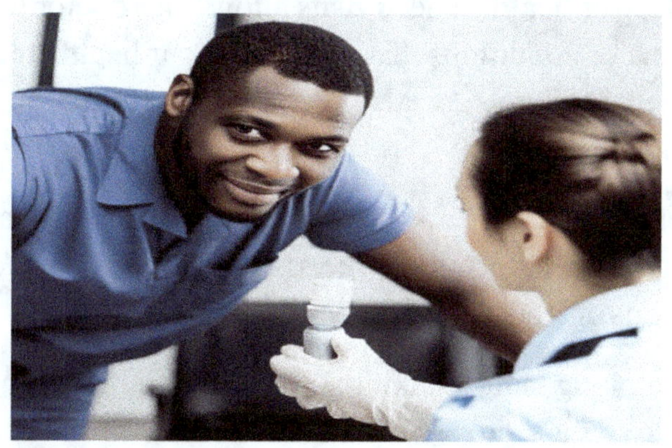

Maintaining good reproductive health is essential for men of all ages. In this chapter, we will discuss the importance of men's reproductive health and provide tips on how to maintain good reproductive health. We will also provide an overview of different reproductive health issues that men may face, such as infertility and prostate health. Additionally, we will discuss the importance of regular check-ups and screenings. We will also provide a list of resources for men who may be struggling with reproductive health issues.

1. Stay informed and up to date on reproductive health: Men should be proactive when it comes to taking care of their reproductive health. Reading books, asking doctors questions, and doing online research are all good ways to stay informed.

2. Practice safe sex: To protect themselves from potentially harmful infections, men should always practice safe sex. This involves

using condoms or other forms of contraception every time they engage in sexual activity.

3. Perform regular self-exams: Men should get in the habit of performing regular self-examinations, as this can help them stay on top of their reproductive health. Testicular cancer and certain other forms of cancer can be found through regular self-exams.

4. Schedule regular check-ups: Yearly or bi-annual check-ups with a primary care physician or urologist are important for maintaining reproductive health. These visits allow your doctor to check for any problems or conditions that could put your health at risk. Checking Testosterone levels is also very important in optimizing male overall well-being.

5. Eat a balanced diet and exercise: Eating healthy and exercising regularly can help reduce the risk of certain reproductive health conditions, such as erectile dysfunction.

6. Quit smoking and drinking: Smoking and drinking can have a negative impact on reproductive health. Quitting these habits can reduce the risk of certain conditions.

Testosterone levels are an important indicator of men's reproductive health. Low testosterone levels can lead to a range of symptoms, such as weight gain, low libido, fatigue, and even memory issues. To ensure adequate testosterone levels, regular checkups and screenings are essential. During these screenings, a qualified healthcare provider can measure and evaluate a man's testosterone levels and develop a strategy for maintaining them.

The first step to checking testosterone levels is ordering a blood test. During this test, healthcare providers will take a sample of blood and measure the amount of testosterone in it. Results from this test can be used to evaluate hormone levels and determine if hormone therapy is necessary.

In addition to regular checkups, there are certain lifestyle factors that can influence testosterone levels. Eating a healthy diet, getting regular exercise, and avoiding excessive alcohol intake are all important for maintaining appropriate hormone levels. Additionally, men should ensure that they are getting sufficient sleep and managing their stress to optimize testosterone levels.

1. Low testosterone can lead to impaired cognitive function, mood changes, fatigue, reduced muscle mass, poor libido, decreased body hair, gynecomastia (breast enlargement), difficulty concentrating, erectile dysfunction, and reduced bone density.

2. The benefits of treatment depend on the cause but can include increased energy and libido, an improved sense of well-being, better muscle, and bone health, improved cognitive function, and a better cardiovascular system. Treatment may also help reduce negative side effects such as gynecomastia and erectile dysfunction. Some studies have suggested that testosterone therapy may even enhance longevity.

3. Testosterone therapy can also provide life-altering physical and psychological benefits. Improved mental clarity, increased libido, better muscle tone, and improved body composition can all be among the positive outcomes of treatment. Additionally, some men see increases in motivation and self-esteem when receiving regular testosterone therapy.

Lastly, there are several resources available to men who may be struggling with testosterone levels. Consulting with a doctor is the best place to start to identify the underlying cause and develop a plan of action. Additionally, there are several educational materials and support groups are available to provide additional information and resources.

Helpful Websites:

- ASRM.org

- ProstateCancerFoundation.org

- MensHealthNetwork.org

CHAPTER 12
MEN'S SKIN HEALTH

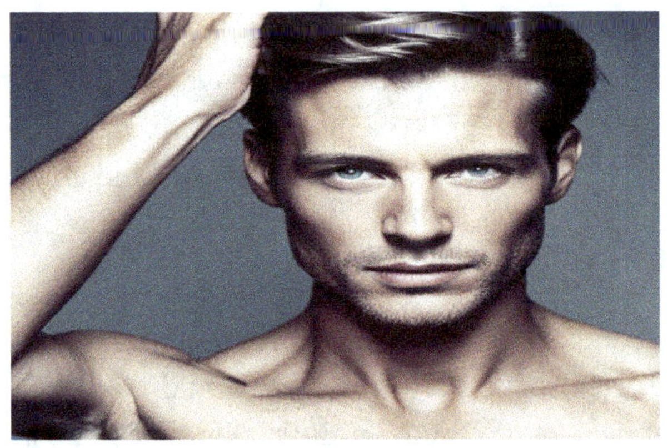

Maintaining good skin health is essential for men of all ages, not only to look and feel good but for overall well-being. To prevent skin health issues such as skin cancer and acne, it is important to practice good habits such as protecting your skin from the sun with sunscreen and protective clothing, eating a healthy diet, avoiding smoking, and washing your skin with mild, moisturizing cleansers. Additionally, regular check-ups and screenings with a dermatologist are key to identifying any skin changes that could signal potential problems or health concerns. Finally, there are also many resources available for men who may be struggling with skin health issues, including accessible and affordable health care, online resources, and support network.

To examine yourself for good skin health and detect skin cancer:

1. Become familiar with your skin's normal appearance. Take note of any moles, freckles, and other marks that may be present.

2. Examine your skin for any changes in texture or color. Pay close attention to your face, scalp, neck, ears, chest, back, and any other areas that can't be easily seen.

3. Check for any new or unusual moles. Look for ones that are significantly different in size, shape, color, or texture from other moles you have.

4. Be aware of any growths that are dark in color, have a mixed color pattern, or have an irregular border.

5. Monitor existing moles for any changes in shape, size, or color. Be aware of any moles that are growing, bleeding, or changing in any unusual way.

6. Look for any abnormal pains or itchy spots.

If you notice any changes or abnormalities, contact your doctor for a full skin assessment.

Skin Self-examination.

Regular skin checks are crucial self-care for men, as skin cancer, including melanoma, affects both genders. Here's a simplified guide to conducting a thorough skin examination:

Choose an appropriate setting: Ensure you have proper lighting, a full-length mirror, and a handheld mirror to examine hard-to-see areas like your back and scalp.

Inspect your entire body: Begin with your face—nose, lips, mouth, and ears—followed by your scalp, neck, chest, arms and underarms. Check hands, fingers, and nails before moving on to your torso, back, buttocks, and genital area. Finish with legs, tops of feet, between toes and soles of feet.

Look for skin irregularities: Monitor moles, freckles, or other skin growths for changes by using the ABCDE rule:

- **Asymmetry:** Check if the mole has differing halves.

- **Border:** Examine for uneven or unclear boundaries.

- **Color:** Look for color variations or multiple colors within a mole.

- **Diameter:** Assess if the mole is more than 6 millimeters (about pencil eraser size).

- **Evolution:** Observe alterations in size, shape or color and any itching, bleeding, or crusting.

Watch for additional skin anomalies: Apart from moles, check for new growths, unhealing sores or areas where the skin appears different from its surroundings like red scaly patches or shiny nodules.

Consult a professional: If you find concerning changes during your self-exam, seek evaluation from a dermatologist or healthcare specialist. Accurate diagnosis and timely treatment are crucial when needed.

Reduce risk.

To lower the risk of skin cancer, it is important to take sun-safe measures and follow a healthy lifestyle. Here are some tips to help avoid skin cancer:

1. Limit Sun Exposure: Stay away from the sun, especially during peak hours when the sun's rays are the strongest, typically between 10 am and 4 pm. Seek shade whenever possible, particularly during midday hours.

2. Cover Up: Cover your skin with loose-fitting, lightweight clothing that provides a physical barrier against the sun's harmful ultraviolet (UV) rays. Wear long sleeves, long pants, wide-brimmed hats, and sunglasses with UV protection.

3. Apply Sunscreen: Use a broad-spectrum sunscreen with an SPF of 30 or higher. Apply generously to all exposed skin, including the face, neck, ears, and hands. Reapply every two hours or more frequently if you're swimming or sweating.

4. Avoid Tanning Beds: They emit UV radiation that can increase the risk of skin cancer.

5. Reflection: Water, sand, snow, and concrete can reflect and intensify the sun's rays. Take extra precautions when you're in these environments.

6. UV Index: Check the daily UV index, which provides information about the strength of UV radiation in your area. Plan outdoor activities accordingly and take appropriate sun protection measures.

7. Self-examinations: Conduct skin self-examinations to monitor your skin for changes or abnormalities. Report concerns a healthcare professional.

8. Professional skin exams: Schedule appointments with a dermatologist for skin examinations. Get insights on early detection and prevention of potential skin cancer risks.

9. Prevent Sunburns: Sunburns increase the risk of skin cancer. Seek shade and wear sun-protective clothing to avoid sunburn.

10. Healthy Lifestyle: Eat a balanced diet rich in fruits, vegetables, and antioxidants. Avoid smoking and limit alcohol consumption, they are linked to increased risk of skin cancer.

Remember, skin cancer prevention is achievable, and through these measures, you can significantly reduce your risk. Stay sun-safe, monitor your skin and consult healthcare professionals for guidance.

Helpful Websites:

- SkinCancer.org

- AAD.org

- Acne.org

CHAPTER 13
MEN'S DENTAL HEALTH

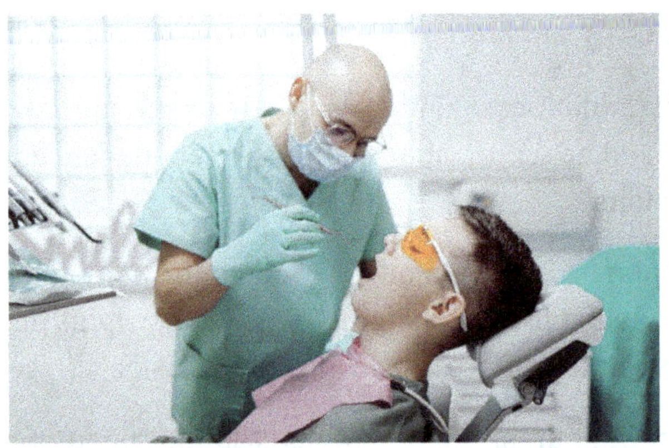

Dental health is an essential aspect of overall health. In this chapter, we will discuss the importance of men's dental health and provide tips on how to maintain good dental health. We will also provide an in-depth look at different dental health issues that men may face, such as gum disease and oral cancer. Additionally, we will discuss the importance of regular check-ups and screenings.

Maintaining good dental health is essential for men of all ages. In this chapter, we will discuss the importance of men's dental health and provide tips on how to maintain good dental health. We will also provide an in-depth look at different dental health issues that men may face, such as gum disease and oral cancer. Additionally, we will discuss the importance of regular check-ups and screenings. We will also provide a list of resources for men who may be struggling with dental health issues.

Poor oral hygiene has been linked to several diseases that affect men's health, including heart and lung diseases, stroke, and diabetes.

1. Poor oral hygiene can increase the risk of cardiovascular disease because bacteria in the mouth can enter the bloodstream and cause inflammation.

2. Poor oral hygiene is associated with a higher risk of developing type 2 diabetes because oral bacteria can enter the bloodstream and disrupt glucose metabolism.

3. Poor oral hygiene may increase the risk of pulmonary infections because harmful oral bacteria can be inhaled into the lungs, causing inflammation and infection.

4. Poor oral hygiene increases the risk of stroke as plaque buildup in the arteries can lead to blockages, resulting in a stroke.

Helpful Websites:

- ADA.org

- MouthHealthy.org

- OralCancerFoundation.org

CHAPTER 14
RED PILL STANDARDS

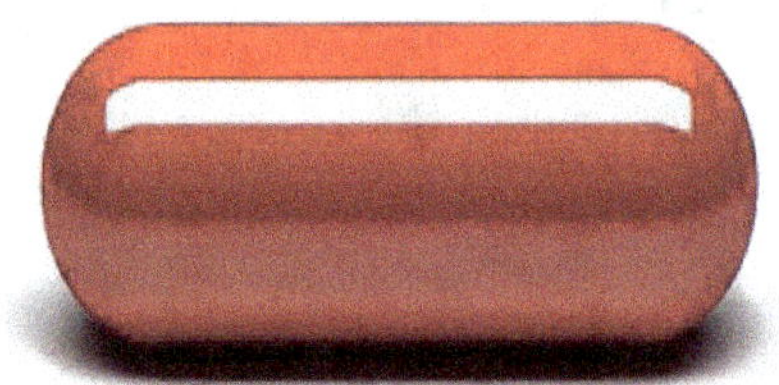

1. Develop a positive attitude towards money management and wealth planning.

2. Make a meaningful effort to build meaningful and loving relationships.

3. Take time for yourself to enjoy and explore hobbies and interests.

4. Balance your work, personal, and family life for a more positive outcome.

5. Priorities self-care and emotional well-being.

6. Spend time in nature to appreciate its beauty and wonder or find your inner beast.

7. Develop better communication and negotiation skills.

8. Invest in yourself through education, skills development, and

furthering your career.

9. Enhance joy and enthusiasm for life through music, art, and literature.

10. Strengthen self-confidence by taking part in activities that promote growth and well-being.

1. Develop a Positive Attitude Towards Money Management and Wealth Planning

Having a positive attitude towards money management and wealth planning is essential to finding financial security and building wealth. This means having a realistic approach to setting goals, understanding the power of compound interest, having a savings plan, and investing wisely.

Step 1: Set goals.

Creating short, medium, and long-term financial goals is the first step to having a positive attitude toward money. Write these goals down and take time to analyze why they are important to you. Consider taking a personal finance course or obtaining advice from a financial advisor to help you stay on track.

Step 2: Understand compound interest.

Compound interest is the additional interest earned on the contents of the original capital investment. It is important to understand that the longer the money is kept in an account, the more interest will accumulate. Consider starting a savings plan to take advantage of compound interest and plan for longer-term goals.

Step 3: Have a savings plan.

A savings plan not only considers compound interest but also helps you save money for a goal or emergency fund. Start by identifying a percentage of your monthly income that can be put towards savings and set this money aside. This could include setting up an automatic savings bank transfer or investing in a high-interest savings account.

Step 4: Invest wisely.

Investing is one of the best ways to see financial returns. It's important to understand that investing carries risk so research the different asset classes and act with caution. Consider investing in stocks, bonds, mutual funds, and ETFs (exchange-traded funds).

Having a positive attitude towards money management and wealth planning is essential to accessing and streamlining your financial goals. It requires discipline, research, and education to make wise money decisions, build wealth, and create a secure financial future.

2. Make a Meaningful Effort to Build Meaningful and Loving Relationships

Relationships are essential to a happy life. Whether it's family, friends, or romantic relationships, making a meaningful effort to strengthen these connections is vital to creating a fulfilled life.

Step 1: Invest quality time.

The best way to build meaningful relationships is to invest quality time. Whether it's a family member or a friend, take time to do something enjoyable together. Spend time catching up on each other's lives, share an experience, or create new memories.

Step 2: Be open and communicative.

Be open and communicative about your thoughts and feelings to build strong connections. Show them that you trust them to listen and support you. Sharing experiences and showing vulnerability is essential to building meaningful relationships with people.

Step 3: Listen without judgment.

We can learn a lot from listening to other people's stories. Show that you are engaged and attentive by listening without judgment. This helps create an environment of safety and support and encourages more meaningful conversations.

Step 4: Offer support and encouragement.

Offer support and encouragement to those around you. It's important to be there for them in times of difficulty and to celebrate their successes. This creates a good foundation of trust and fosters strong relationships.

Making a meaningful effort to build relationships is essential to creating a happy and fulfilling life. It's important to invest time in the important people in your life and show them that you care about them.

3. Take Time for Yourself to Enjoy and Explore Hobbies and Interests

Having hobbies and interests to explore is a great way to give our lives more meaning. Taking time for ourselves to try new activities and pursue our passions can help us to find joy and satisfaction.

Step 1: Identify Interests

The first step to creating time to explore our hobbies is to identify what interests us. Whether it's reading, photography, hiking, cooking, or anything else, try to identify activities that bring you joy and collect information on each interest.

Step 2: Explore Different Activities

Once you have identified interests, it's time to start exploring them. Consider visiting a nearby public library, museum, gallery, or national park to start. To begin, try activities which are free or low-cost.

Step 3: Invest in Learning

Investing in learning a skill or interest can help to deepen our understanding and enjoyment. Whether it's taking a cooking class or joining a photography course, researching ways to gain more knowledge can help to hone our skills and increase our enjoyment.

Step 4: Take Time for Yourself

Once you've identified your interests and started exploring them, be sure to take time for yourself to enjoy them. Make sure to plan rest days to reflect and relax. This helps to keep your activities enjoyable and allows for personal growth.

4. Balance your work, personal, and family life for a more positive outcome

Work-life balance for men emphasizes the importance of having a well-balanced life that considers work, personal, and family life. It encourages men to understand that family life is important even if they have a demanding job. As such, men should strive to maintain an appropriate balance between their life at work, their personal life, and their home life to have a more positive outcome from their overall lifestyle.

For example, men should strive to maintain a healthy relationship with their family members, without sacrificing their work or personal goals. This could include regularly attending family gatherings, making time for quality family time, and being present for important life events.

In addition, men should prioritize taking time for themselves to relax and enjoy hobbies. This could be as simple as setting aside time to play a sport, enjoying nature, meeting up with friends, or just taking time out to reflect.

Men should also invest in themselves through education, skills development, and furthering their careers. This could involve taking part in professional development workshops, taking online classes to increase knowledge, attempting new tasks or responsibilities at work, or even starting their own business.

Finally, men should learn to prioritize self-care and emotional well-being. This could involve exercising, eating healthy, getting enough rest, meditating, and taking care of their physical and mental health. It is important to practice activities that bring about joy and enthusiasm for life, such as taking walks, listening to music, painting, reading, or exploring the outdoors.

5. Priorities self-care and emotional well-being.

By implementing these strategies, men can work towards achieving a balanced life that prioritizes work, personal goals, and family time. Doing so can produce better outcomes for their work and personal life while also strengthening relationships and improving overall well-being.

Prioritizing self-care and emotional well-being is an essential component of an empowerment mindset for men. Self-care includes activities such as regular exercise, eating healthy and nutritious meals, getting enough sleep, and taking time for yourself each day. This can involve taking a bath, going for a jog, or simply taking time to meditate and clear your mind.

Additionally, it is important to make your emotional well-being a priority. Managing stress, practicing acceptance of yourself and others, and communicating openly are all actions that enable greater emotional stability and resilience. This means actively seeking out counseling, if necessary, as well as taking part in activities that make you feel relaxed and content such as Yoga or mindfulness meditation.

These steps, when taken together, create a strong foundation for personal growth and empowerment. In addition to improving your overall health and well-being, these activities also encourage greater self-awareness and self-confidence; helping you to recognize the strengths and potential that you may have been overlooking. Overall, prioritizing self-care and emotional well-being plays a key role in successfully developing an empowerment mindset for men.

"You can achieve greatness when you prioritize your self-care and emotional well-being. Taking the time to focus on yourself and practice acceptance of yourself and others is the key to unlocking the best version of yourself. By investing in your physical and mental health, you can develop a strong sense of self-worth and self-confidence that will open the doors to limitless possibilities. Embrace your power and potential and reach for newfound heights in life." CA

6. Empowering Mindset

To have an empowering mindset and truly own your power, it is important to spend time in nature and appreciate its beauty and wonders. Nature can heal, inspire, and bring peace and harmony to the soul. It can provide a perfect environment for relaxation, mindfulness, and self-reflection.

For example, taking a walk in the park or going for a hike in the hills can help men to slow down, be in the present moment, and gain a newfound appreciation for the natural world. Not only can it be a great source of physical exercise, but it is also a great way to connect with yourself and admire the beauty around you without any distractions.

Other activities in nature that you could pursue to further your empowerment are outdoor sports, such as biking, running, kayaking, and fishing. Enjoying activities in nature can help you reset and re-charge while actively appreciating the beauty of nature. It is a great way to unplug from the busyness of life and reconnect with yourself. Participating in activities such as these can help you to build self-confidence and self-esteem while also giving you a greater appreciation for the beauty and grandeur of the natural world.

"Men, the time has come to recognize and own your power. Empowerment starts with taking time for yourself and appreciating the beauty of nature. Taking a slow walk in the park, a hike in the woods, or a bike ride outdoors can help to reset your mind and inspire you. Fishing, kayaking, and other outdoor sports can also help to boost confidence and self-esteem. Make taking care of yourself a priority and remember that nature can be a great source of relaxation and reflection. Embrace the beauty of the natural world and find the power and strength within yourself to succeed." CA

7. Develop better communication and negotiation skills

Understanding and honing communication and negotiation skills are tremendously important for any individual or group that wishes to achieve great outcomes. A powerful man needs to have the ability to effectively make his point and determine what is most important, both verbally and in writing.

One example to acquire better communication and negotiation skills is to observe successful people in various fields and emulate them. Say, if a person wants to pursue a career in sales, he should observe the best salespersons in the industry and take note of the tactics and strategies they use to close deals.

Another example to acquire better communication and negotiation skills is to practice with friends and family. By giving and receiving constructive feedback, people can develop an understanding of their communication habits and weaknesses. Moreover, gaining the practice and confidence of communicating with people close to you will make it easier to effectively negotiate in public spaces.

Following some of these steps, it's not only possible to become more aware of existing boundaries and limitations, but also how to successfully navigate them to come out on top. A powerful man needs to be able to successfully get his points across and navigate difficult conversations. With the right balance of knowledge and practice, communication and negotiation ideologies can be applied in a successful way.

8. Investing in yourself through education, skills development, and furthering your career

Investing in yourself through education, skills development, and furthering your career are other ways to elevate yourself. This is an essential part of becoming a powerful man. Education is key to expanding one's mind and learning new skills and ways of thinking. It is important to build knowledge and above all, strive for excellence in whatever field you are in. Learn from other powerful men and mimic their way of life and how they navigate the world. Skills development equips one with strong technical and communication skills, which enable them to be productive and effective team players. They also enable one to be creative and open-minded to try new ideas and approaches. Furthering one's career is also essential to becoming a powerful man. This involves actively seeking out opportunities to demonstrate one's abilities, ambitions, and determination. It also involves continuously taking on new projects, challenges, and tasks to demonstrate competency in one's field and show the capability to take on greater and more complex roles.

Ultimately a powerful man should also actively seek out networking opportunities to build connections within their industry and enhance their reputation and credibility.

Powerful Moves:

1. Practice positive affirmations and self-talk.

2. Find a mentor or role model.

3. Explore different cultures and broaden your horizons.

4. Exercise regularly and eat a healthy diet.

5. Maintain a gratitude journal or practice gratitude meditation.

6. Foster a creative outlet - painting, drawing, sculpting, etc.

7. Participate in activities that bring joy - cooking, theatre, gaming, etc.

8. Get enough sleep and practice mindful relaxation.

9. Spend time with animals and nature.

10. Develop your spiritual side and try out different spiritual practices.

11. Get involved in volunteer work in the community.

12. Challenge yourself to learn a new skill.

13. Travel and become a tourist in your own city.

14. Upgrade your wardrobe and practice self-care.

Practice Positive Affirmations and Self-talk

Practicing positive affirmations and self-talk is an important tool to help boost your self-confidence and self-belief. Research has shown that replacing negative thought patterns with positive ones can influence our overall happiness and well-being.

Step 1: Identify Self-Limiting Beliefs

The first step is to identify any negative self-talk or self-limiting beliefs that may be preventing you from being happy. This could include phrases such as "I'm not good enough" and "I can't do it". Once you are aware of any limiting beliefs, it will be easier to replace them with positive affirmations.

Step 2: Create Positive Affirmations

Now it's time to create positive affirmations using words that are meaningful and motivating. Some powerful affirmations include "I am enough", "I am capable and strong", and "I have the power to create change". You can also create affirmations that are specific to your goals or desires.

Step 3: Repeat Daily

Once you have identified any negative thought patterns and created positive affirmations, repeat them to yourself each day. Repeat them out loud, in front of a mirror, or look at them on a note or on your phone. This helps to ensure that the affirmations become internalized and start to manifest in your life.

Practicing positive affirmations is a great way to reprogram your subconscious and create happiness and positivity in your life. With regular repetition, you can start to witness real changes in terms of motivation and confidence.

Find a Mentor or Role Model

Step 1: Find Someone You Admire

The first step is to find someone you admire and aspire to emulate. This could be a mentor, a friend, a famous figure, or anyone who resonates with you. Make sure to research and observe their qualities, their values, and their successes.

Step 2: Make Connections

If possible, take steps to build a relationship with this person or find out if they offer mentorship. Reach out to them through social media, make contact in person, or join a group or class where they are present. This helps to create an environment of trust and support which allows you to learn from and understand each other.

Step 3: Schedule Meetings

Once you have reached out to the mentor or role model, it is important to schedule regular meetings. This could be weekly or bi-weekly over Skype, phone, or in person. Make sure to be organized and prepared for each meeting and think of questions or topics you'd like to discuss.

Step 4: Take Action

The most important step is to act and try to apply the knowledge your mentor or role model is sharing. Having a mentor or role model will be of no use if you do not act on their advice and apply it to your own life.

Connecting with a mentor or role model can be a great way to gain motivation and gain valuable knowledge from someone with experience. It helps to build relationships and create an environment of trust and support that can lead to personal growth and happiness.

Explore Different Cultures and Broaden Your Horizons

Exploring cultures different from your own can be a great way to open yourself up to new perspectives, experiences, and ideas. It also helps to build empathy and understanding and can help to create a sense of connectedness within the world.

Step 1: Research

The first step is to research different cultures, religions, and regions around the world. This can be done through reading books, accessing online resources, or traveling if you are able to do so. Use your research to understand the different beliefs and traditions of the culture you are exploring.

Step 2: Talk to People

Reaching out to people who come from different cultural backgrounds is a great way to gain insight and gain a deeper understanding of the culture. This could be done by talking to people in person, or by joining online communities or forums.

Step 3: Practice Sensitivity and Respect

Make sure to always practice sensitivity and respect when discussing or exploring different cultures. Remember that your perspective is not the only one and try to take small steps to learn more about other cultures and their traditions.

Step 4: Immerse Yourself

If possible, try to take part in different cultural activities such as attending cultural events, festivals, or workshops. This can be a great way to learn more about a culture first-hand and to experience different values and traditions.

Exploring different cultures and broadening your horizons can be a great way to gain perspective, empathy, and understanding of the world. It can also help to create a more tolerant and accepting outlook which can lead to greater well-being and happiness.

"Taking time for yourself to enjoy and explore hobbies and interests is a great way to bring more satisfaction and joy into your life. Identifying your interests and taking time to enjoy and expand your knowledge of them can help you find fulfillment and appreciation in your life."

Exercise and fun alternatives to exercise

One positive lifestyle adjustment a man can make to enhance self-happiness is to exercise regularly. This can include activities such as running, jogging, hiking, swimming, or basketball, to name a few. Exercise releases endorphins, which provide an emotional boost, help reduce stress, and enhance overall well-being. Regular exercise can also help build strong bones, improve the quality of sleep, increase energy, and boost self-esteem. Additionally, participating in high-intensity interval training (H.I.I.T.) for short durations can also be beneficial for conditioning your body and improving energy levels.

Another positive lifestyle adjustment men can make to enhance self-happiness is to eat a healthy diet. This can include incorporating more fruits and vegetables into your diet and avoiding processed foods. Eating healthy has the potential to help improve mood and physical health, increase energy, and give you more mental clarity. Eating healthy can also involve adopting various other diets, such as vegetarian, vegan, keto, or the Mediterranean diet.

Men can increase their self-happiness by spending time outdoors. Going outdoors can help reduce stress, clear the mind, and increase happiness. Activities such as hiking, rock climbing, trekking, camping, and other outdoor adventure sports can help increase endorphin production, reduce anxiety, and help with connecting with nature. Taking breaks from technology and logging off from social media can also help to reduce stress and worry.

Exercise can have a tremendously positive effect on a person's self-esteem and confidence in their own worthiness, and ultimately their attractiveness to the opposite sex. Regular physical exercise can lead to improved body composition, improved physical coordination, and stamina where it counts, as well as an overall sense of accomplishment and improved self-image. People who exercise often have increased levels of testosterone, which can further boost their sense of confidence and self-worth. Regular exercise not only helps people feel better about themselves and look better physically but can also enable them to perform better in social situations and show off their great qualities to the opposite sex more effectively.

Alternatives to exercise

1. Dance: Not only is it a great way to get your heart rate up, but it is also a fun and creative way to move your body while listening to music.

2. Yoga: Whether you're practicing traditional poses or doing your own flow, yoga is a great way to stay active and increase flexibility.

3. Tai Chi: This low-impact exercise is great for reducing stress and improving balance.

4. Parkour: This increasingly popular physical activity can help test your strength, agility, and coordination.

5. Jump Rope: This activity requires no equipment and can be done both indoors and outdoors.

6. Frisbee: This game can be played with a group of friends or solo, making it an excellent way to stay socially active while also exercising.

7. Rock Climbing: Whether you're scaling a rock wall or bouldering outdoors, rock climbing is a great way to stay physically active.

8. Kayaking: This activity is great for testing your strength and balance while also enjoying the beauty of nature.

9. Tour Skating: This activity involves skating up and down hills on a longboard or inline skates while enjoying a scenic tour.

10. Skateboarding: This popular activity is a great way to express your creative side and stay active.

Practicing Gratitude and Appreciation

Practicing gratitude and appreciation is an important part of leading a happy and fulfilled life. Practicing gratitude and appreciation can help to foster more positive emotions and attitudes which can, in turn, lead to improved relationships, more meaningful experiences, and even better physical health. Men can incorporate gratitude and appreciation into their lives by taking the time to appreciate what they have in the present moment and taking time to develop meaningful relationships and experiences.

Some steps that men can take to incorporate gratitude and appreciation into their lives include:

- Taking the time to write down three to five things that they are grateful for each day. This can help to remind them of the blessings they have in life.

- Making an effort to be kind and give back to their communities. This can include volunteering their time or donating money to causes they believe in.

- Spending time with the people they care about and taking the time to appreciate the relationships in their lives.

- Nurturing their passions and talents. Taking the time to engage in meaningful activities can help to foster a sense of appreciation for the joys in life.

- Practicing self-care. Taking breaks from time to time can help men to appreciate all that they do and help them to find balance.

- Showing compassion. Practicing self-compassion can help men to be more understanding and empathetic towards themselves and others.

Some helpful links and resources for learning more about practical tools for developing and incorporating gratitude and appreciation into one's life include:

- Gratitude Worksheets from The Feel-Good Guide: https://imjohnhopkins.com/the-feel-good-guide/gratitude-worksheets/

- Appreciating the Good in Your Life from The Huffington Post: http://www.huffingtonpost.com/jeff-haden/appreciate-the-good-in-you_b_9181704.html

- 18 Ways to Keep Gratitude Alive from Salute Magazine: http://www.salute-magazine.com/18-ways-to-keep-gratitude-alive/

- Compassion-Focused Therapy from the Centre for Applied Compassion: https://centreforcompassion.com/what-is-compassion-focused-therapy/

Foster a Creative Outlet

Finding creative outlets is one of the most important and effective things men can do to enhance self-happiness. This can take many forms such as painting, drawing, sculpting, music, gardening, theater, and more. Having something creative to work on can be a great way to reduce stress and relax. Try out different possibilities until you find something that resonates with you.

Alternatives

- Photography

- Woodworking

- Pottery and ceramics

- Furniture repair and restoration

- Video production and editing

- Grilling on the woods

- Graphic design and illustration

- Drawing mandalas

- Gardening

- Creating and assembling models

Participate in Activities that Bring Joy

One of the most proactive steps that men can take to enhance their self-happiness is to pursue activities that bring them joy. There are countless activities that can be uplifting and positive, from cooking, baking, gardening, and woodworking to theatre, music, filmmaking, and gaming.

Outdoor grilling can bring a sense of belonging and collaboration, as working with others or attempting challenging recipes can be rewarding and fun. Exercising can bring lasting energy, improved sleep, and mental clarity, which often translates into greater productivity and well-being.

Gardening and woodworking can be satisfying in different ways- maintaining a garden can be a relaxing, meditative activity, while the woodwork can leverage creative outlets and even give tangible results. Practicing theatre, (such as singing, dancing, acting), creating and producing music, films, and video games can provide an escape and an escape and an outlet for self-expression.

No matter which activities a man chooses to pursue, doing something that brings joy can be one of the most positive adjustments that one can make for their overall well-being and happiness.

Get back to nature

Spend time with animals and nature: To enhance self-happiness, men should take some time each day to reconnect with nature and animals. This could mean taking a walk in a park or forest and noticing the rugged environment, spending time at the zoo and connecting with the animals and getting your inner beast back.

Not only does being connected to the natural world help us stay grounded, but it can also boost our happiness and mental health. Studies have reported that spending time in nature can reduce stress, improve concentration, and relieve symptoms of depression. Animals provide companionship and unconditional love and offer many physical and mental health benefits such as decreasing stress and blood pressure and increasing communication and self-discipline.

If engaging with animals and nature is not possible due to the current situation, there are still plenty of positive lifestyle adjustments that men can make such as watching nature documentaries, planting a home garden, and joining online forums to discuss environmental issues. Additionally, meditating and practicing mindfulness can help men stay connected to the present moment and the beauty of nature surrounding them.

Speak to your soul

Speaking of spiritual practices, men can make positive lifestyle adjustments to enhance self-happiness by incorporating different types of spiritual practices into their lives. This could include activities such as yoga, meditation, prayer, Buddhist mindfulness exercises, and visualization.

Yoga can help reduce stress, improve mental clarity, and cultivate balance. Through yoga, men can learn to quiet their minds and find peace. It can also help build strength, coordination, and discipline by combining physical poses with mindful breathing.

Meditation is a great way to center oneself and focus on self-improvement. It can help relax the body and ease the mind, which is essential for emotional well-being. During meditation, it's important to focus on positive thinking, allowing your thoughts to flow freely without judgment.

Prayer can also be a source of comfort and solace. By setting aside dedicated time for prayer, men can reflect on their lives and find serenity. Praying to a higher power allows men to contemplate life's uncertainties as well as practice humility and gratitude.

Buddhist mindfulness exercises can help men observe their thoughts and feelings, recognize patterns in their behavior, and gain insight into their reactions and responses. By observing their emotions without judgment, men can separate themselves from them and see them objectively.

Visualization is a great way to imagine a future that is full of possibilities and growth. Men can use visualization to explore deeply held dreams, goals, and aspirations. Visualization can help men tap into their innermost desires and take steps to achieve them.

Overall, incorporating a variety of spiritual practices into your life can open many different pathways to emotional well-being. Men can find the tools necessary to develop inner strength and become their happiest selves.

CHAPTER 15
RED PILL MINDSET

Men should maintain a high standard and not settle for mediocrity when it comes to modern women and the right spouse because the type of partner, they choose can drastically shape their future. Choosing a spouse that is not up to your standards can have negative impacts on your life, such as making it more difficult to achieve your goals, hampering your earnings potential, and potentially making it harder for you to sustain healthy relationships. When it comes to finding a partner, men should demand quality to keep up with modern women's standards and ensure that they find a person that can help them grow and live happily.

Having a quality relationship with a modern woman can help a man reach his goals in several ways. Firstly, choosing a partner with similar values and goals can motivate each other to strive to become the best version of themselves. Additionally, with mutual respect and understanding, both partners can provide each other with emotional support and advice when pursuing individual objectives. Their support can range from giving encouragement and being a sounding board to helping to achieve their goals with practical solutions.

Furthermore, a high-quality partner can open your horizon to valuable opportunities and connections. For example, your partner may have access to certain resources or contacts that can help you reach a higher level of success. Additionally, having someone who is driven and passionate about their own life can be an enormous motivation to constantly learn and do more.

Therefore, it is essential for men to not settle for mediocrity when it comes to modern women and the right spouse. By keeping themselves to a high standard and investing time and effort into finding someone with similar values and goals, men can unlock the door to a world of opportunity. This way, they can surround themselves with people who are looking to do great things and have an even greater chance of reaching the goals they set for themselves. These relationships can blossom to create unique and lasting bonds that can help them better their lives overall ,or men who are looking for alternatives to modern women in the West, there are numerous options available. For example, men can look to more traditional societies, such as those found in parts of Asia or South America. In these cultures, it is often more common for men and women to enter marriage or relationships based on more archaic values and expectations of the roles of men and women.

In addition, men can look to certain religious communities as an alternative. Depending on the region or group, the rules for courtship and dating may be quite different from what is found in the modern societies of the West. For example, many Islamic marriages are organized via the families of the bride and groom without requiring the couple to have met prior to the wedding.

Men can also explore different forms of polyamory as an alternative. Polyamory is defined as the practice of loving or being committed to more than one person at the same time. This could include being part of a throuple, a foursome, or just having two partners at once. While polyamory is still practiced in a relatively small percentage of the population, it is becoming increasingly more accepted and accepted in the mainstream.

The world is your playground:

(Before traveling to other countries please know their laws and regulation)

Traveling to other countries can be a great way to enhance self-happiness by expanding one's horizons and challenging one to step out of their comfort zone. Countries such as India and Morocco offer an experience like no other. In India, men can explore the vibrant culture, incredible food, and remarkable architecture, all while absorbing the unmatched energy of the bustling cities. Morocco is a perfect spot for those who love adventure and exploring the great outdoors as there are numerous deserts, mountains, and beaches to explore. Aside from the great sightseeing opportunities, men can meet and interact with women who are appreciative of men. In some countries, like China and Japan, women are still expected to adhere to rigid gender roles and can sometimes come off as distant or uninterested. However, in countries like India and Morocco, women are usually more open to meeting and engaging with men from outside their culture, and there is more mutual respect and appreciation between men and women. Additionally, there are plenty of beautiful landscapes, historic sites, and activities to take part in while exploring these countries such as yoga activities, exploring remote villages, spas, and nearby beaches. With all, men can really benefit from traveling to other countries as it provides them with the opportunity to expand their horizons, meet new people, and gain a greater sense of self-happiness.

Traditional women in these countries differ in terms of their cultural roles and expectations. In India, women are typically expected to be strong, and devoted, and to remain focused on family and home responsibilities. They are also expected to take a more conservative approach to life, although this is becoming less rigid, especially among the younger generations. In Morocco, women are typically the main caretakers of the home and may wear traditional clothing to signify their religious beliefs. Women are also expected to take on duties such as looking after the family's children and tending to the household chores. In Thailand, women are expected to be obedient and respectful, as well as good at cooking and taking care of the home. Women are also expected to adhere to traditional gender norms and are not usually encouraged to pursue higher education or careers. In Kenya, women are guardians of traditional values and are considered primary caregivers for children. Women are also typically expected to marry at an early age and perform domestic duties such as cooking and cleaning. In Brazil, women are expected to take on a more traditional role in the home, such as raising children and caring for the family. However, Brazil has seen an increase in women achieving higher levels of education and pursuing successful careers. All in all, traditional women in these countries are often given certain expectations and roles by their societies, which they are expected to live up to.

Get the woman you want:

It is not possible to get any woman you want. At the end of the day, it's up to the woman to decide whether she's interested in you. The best thing you can do is focus on being the best version of yourself, building your confidence, and developing strong social skills. Putting yourself out there and engaging in meaningful conversations is the best way to attract someone who is compatible with you.

Put in the effort to create a good impression- This means smiling, making eye contact, and maintaining positive body language. Act with self-confidence and show that you are an interesting and reliable person.

Be genuine- Women can easily spot a disingenuous person. Therefore, being genuine and authentic in your interactions will make you stand out and make a real connection in a genuine way.

Be polite- Refrain from crude jokes and language or making negative remarks. Demonstrate good manners and respect the opinion of the woman you're with.

Listen- Be attentive to what the woman is saying and ask her questions about her life. Show interest in what she's telling you and remember the details she's shared with you.

Be positive- Maintaining a positive attitude is essential. Being confident in yourself and having an upbeat outlook on life radiates a sense of passion and joy that can be contagious.

Check out these 12 vacation spots perfect for socializing and meeting new people:

1. Rio de Janeiro, Brazil - www.visitbrasil.com: Vibrant nightlife, beautiful beaches, and an energetic atmosphere.

2. Barcelona, Spain - www.barcelona.cat/en/: Lively street culture, bustling bars, and stunning architecture.

3. Bali, Indonesia - www.indonesia.travel/gb/en/home: Gorgeous beaches, relaxation, and a vibrant nightlife scene.

4. Stockholm, Sweden - www.visitstockholm.com: Charming city with lively nightlife, cultural events, and progressive atmosphere.

5. Buenos Aires, Argentina - www.buenosaires.gob.ar/turismo/en: Tango culture, exciting nightlife, and passionate locals.

6. Cape Town, South Africa - www.capetown.travel: Stunning landscapes, vibrant culture, and diverse social scenes.

7. Bangkok, Thailand - www.tourismthailand.org/home: Ancient temples, lively street markets, and thriving nightlife.

8. Prague, Czech Republic - www.prague.eu/en: Rich history, beautiful architecture, and lively pub culture.

9. Tel Aviv, Israel - www.visit-tel-aviv.com: Cosmopolitan city with vibrant nightlife and beautiful beaches.

10. Amsterdam, Netherlands - www.iamsterdam.com: Relaxed atmosphere with canal-lined streets and exciting nightlife.

11. Tokyo, Japan - www.gotokyo.org/en: Bustling metropolis offering a unique cultural experience.

12. Lisbon, Portugal - www.visitportugal.com/en: Charming streets with a lively music scene and friendly locals.

It is important to note that traveling to a foreign country carries risks and safety should always be a priority. These destinations still offer fantastic opportunities to socialize and potentially meet single women. Have a great time exploring!

CHAPTER 16
COOK LIKE A CAVEMAN

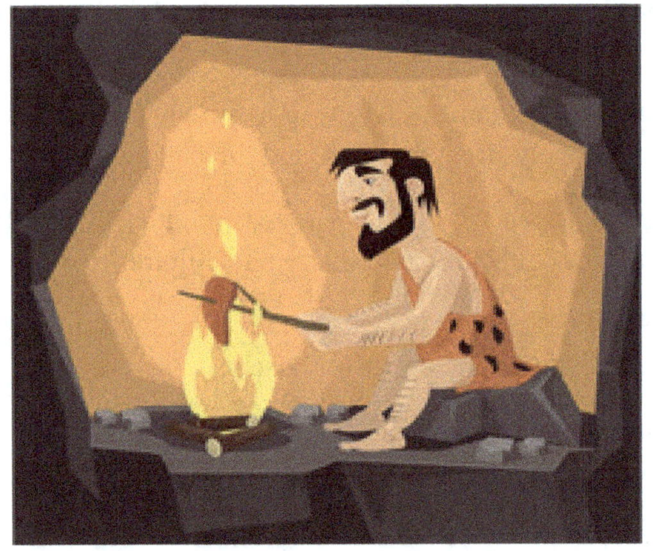

A few manly recipes

Next page

Jamaican jerk chicken: *fire breathing (spicey).*

Ingredients:

- 2 tablespoons light brown sugar
- 2 tablespoons dried thyme
- 1 Scotch bonnet pepper
- 2 tablespoons allspice
- 2 teaspoons sea salt
- 1 teaspoon garlic powder
- 1 teaspoon onion powder
- 2 teaspoons freshly ground black pepper.
- 2 teaspoons ground nutmeg
- 2 tablespoons ground ginger
- ½ teaspoon cayenne pepper
- 4 (8-ounce) boneless and skinless chicken breasts
- ½ cup freshly squeezed lime juice
- 4 tablespoons vegetable oil

Instructions:

1. In a small bowl, whisk together the light brown sugar, thyme, allspice, sea salt, garlic powder, onion powder, black pepper, nutmeg, ground ginger, and cayenne pepper until combined.

2. Place the chicken breasts into a large zip-top bag or shallow bowl. Pour the lime juice over the chicken, followed by the vegetable oil and dry seasoning. Rub the marinade onto the chicken until evenly coated.

3. Cover the bag or bowl and place it into the refrigerator to marinate for at least 1 hour and up to 8 hours. The longer it marinades, the more flavorful it will be.

4. Preheat the grill to medium heat.

5. When it's ready, grill the chicken for 5 to 6 minutes per side, then smoke for 60 minutes at 250°F in a smoker. or bake in the oven at 375 for 35 minutes.

6. Serve with your favorite side dishes and enjoy.

Grilled steak, *Caribbean style*

Ingredients:

- 1 teaspoon of ground allspice

- 1 teaspoon of brown sugar

- 2 tablespoons of olive oil

- 1 clove garlic, chopped.

- 1 teaspoon of ground ginger

- 1 teaspoon of dried thyme

- 1 pinch of ground nutmeg

- 1 teaspoon of ground black pepper

- 1/2 teaspoon of salt

- 1 lb. of steak (such as sirloin or flank steak)

Instructions:

1. Combine allspice, brown sugar, olive oil, garlic, ginger, thyme, nutmeg, and black pepper in a bowl and whisk to combine.

2. Rub the steak with the spice mixture. Cover and let it marinate in the

refrigerator for at least 30 minutes or up to 24 hours.

3. Heat a cast iron or heavy-bottomed skillet over medium-high heat. Add the steak and cook for 4-6 minutes per side (depending on how thick the cut is) for medium.

4. Cover with a lid and let it rest for 5 minutes before slicing and serving.

5. Sprinkle the steak with a pinch of salt and enjoy!

Steak Burritos: *manly size*

Ingredients

- 2 lb flank steak

- 6 burrito-sized flour tortillas

- 2 cups canned refried beans

- 1 cup grated cheese

- 1/2 cup diced onions

- 1/2 cup diced red pepper

- 2 tablespoons olive oil

- 2 tablespoons chili powder

- 1 teaspoon cumin

- 1 teaspoon garlic powder

- 1 teaspoon salt

Instructions

1. Preheat oven to 350°F.

2. Mix together chili powder, cumin, garlic powder and salt in a bowl. Rub mixture onto the flank steak.

3. Heat olive oil in a large skillet over medium-high heat. Add steak and cook for 4-5 minutes per side or until the steak is well-seared.

4. Remove steak from skillet and let rest on a cutting board for 10 minutes.

5. In the same skillet, sauté diced onions and red pepper until softened.

6. Slice steak into thin strips.

7. Heat the refried beans in a medium-sized saucepan or in the microwave.

8. Assemble the burritos by heating each tortilla in a skillet over medium heat for 1 minute per side. Place a few steak strips, refried beans and sautéed onions and peppers in the center of the burrito. Top with a sprinkle of cheese.

9. Roll up the burritos, tucking the ends underneath. Place on a baking sheet and bake in the oven for 10 minutes.

10. Serve hot. Enjoy!

Steak Tacos: *with the beast crunch*

Ingredients:

- 1 pound flank steak (or other cuts of choice)

- 4 cloves garlic, minced

- 1 tablespoon chili powder

- 1 teaspoon ground cumin

- 1 teaspoon smoked paprika

- 1 teaspoon sea salt

- 2 tablespoons olive oil

- 1/4 cup cilantro, chopped

- 12 small soft flour tortillas

- Toppings of choice - guacamole, salsa, diced onion, diced tomato, shredded lettuce, cilantro

Instructions:

1. Start by combining the garlic, chili powder, cumin, smoked paprika, sea salt, and olive oil in a small bowl.

2. Slice the steak into thin strips and place it in a large bowl. Pour the mixture from the small bowl over the steak, making sure to coat it evenly.

3. Heat a large skillet or grill over medium heat. Add the steak strips to the pan and cook for 3 - 4 minutes, or until desired doneness.

4. Transfer the cooked steak to a plate. To assemble the tacos, place some steak strips on a tortilla, top with desired toppings, and sprinkle with cilantro.

5. Serve warm and enjoy!

Catch and cook Shellfish

1. Gather your ingredients: For this recipe, you will need 2 lobsters or crabs, some oil (olive or vegetable oil), some butter, garlic cloves, fresh herbs, and lemons or limes.

2. Build a fire: Use dry wood and kindling and build a fire on the beach. Allow the fire to burn for about 45 minutes.

3. Place Lobsters/Crabs on the Fire: Each lobster or crab should be placed on the fire for approximately 20 minutes per side. The fire should be hot enough that the claws and shells of the lobster/crab become red and charred.

4. Remove Lobsters/Crabs from the Fire: Use tongs or a flat tool to remove the lobster/crab from the fire. Allow to cool for 5 minutes before handling.

5. Remove Shells from Lobsters/Crabs: Use a crab cracker and pliers or knife to remove the claws, legs, and shells from the lobster/crab. Discard shells and set aside chocolate flesh.

6. Prepare Herbs: Finely dice fresh herbs such as parsley or rosemary and set aside for later.

7. Heat a Pan: Heat a cast iron or heavy-bottomed pan over medium heat with 1 tablespoon of oil and 1 tablespoon of butter.

8. Add Garlic and Herbs: Add a few cloves of minced garlic and the chopped herbs. Stir and cook for 1-2 minutes.

9. Add the Lobster/Crab Flesh: Add the lobster/crab flesh to the pan and cook for an additional 4-5 minutes.

10. Add Lemons/Limes: Squeeze fresh lemon or lime juice into the pan and stir.

11. Serve: Remove the pan from the heat and serve the lobster/crab right away. Enjoy!

Herbs and tonics to improve men's vitality and power

- St. John's Wort: St. John's wort is an herb used to support healthy mood balance and can also help support healthy energy levels.

- Ginseng: Studies suggest that ginseng may be beneficial for treating male fertility problems.

- Ashwagandha: Ashwagandha is an adaptogen that helps reduce stress levels and boosts vitality.

- Rhodiola: Rhodiola is an herb that helps to reduce fatigue and improve energy levels.

- Maca: Maca is a Peru botanical that helps to improve libido, energy level, and fertility.

- Tribulus Terrestris: Tribulus Terrestris has been used in traditional

Chinese medicine to improve sexual performance and increase energy levels.

- Horny Goat Weed: Horny goat weed is an herb that is believed to enhance libido, increase sexual stamina, and boost energy levels.

- Astragalus: Astragalus is an adaptogen that helps to relieve stress and fatigue.

- Yohimbe: Yohimbe is an herb that has been used to improve male sexual performance and energy.

- Licorice Root: Licorice root is an herb that has traditionally been used to improve sexual energy and vitality.

- Eleuthero: Eleuthero, also known as Siberian ginseng, has been used to increase energy levels and improve stamina.

- Cistanche: Cistanche is a Chinese herb that may help improve male virility and stamina.

- Shilajit: Shilajit is a Himalayan supplement that can provide a boost of energy and improve mental clarity.

Above all else, it is essential to foster networks of acceptability and mentorship in your industry to grow and reach greater heights. Networking will help you to expand your horizons and become more marketable for job prospects, as well as increase your credentials.

Remember, the journey to becoming a powerful man will take time, dedication, and resilience. It is important to never give up and trust in the process of growing. Every step - even the smallest ones - contributes to your success. Surround yourself with others who can motivate and support you in your journey and never forget to trust in yourself and your abilities no matter what. With a strong work ethic and determination, paired with self-confidence, you can reach the top of the pinnacle and make a strong mark in the world.

Good luck on your journey!

CONCLUSION

In conclusion, men's health is a critical aspect of overall well-being. Maintaining good health is essential for men of all ages, and it is crucial to prioritize your health and well-being to prevent various health issues. This book provides an in-depth look at different aspects of men's health, including nutrition and diet, exercise and fitness, mental health, sexual health, sleep, heart health, cancer support and resources, substance abuse and addiction, men's reproductive health, skin health, and dental health. By understanding the tips and advice provided in this book and utilizing the helpful resources listed, men can maintain good health and live a long and healthy life.

To conclude, every man has the potential to be powerful and reach greater heights with confidence. With strong communication and negotiation skills at your disposal, you can tackle any challenge and conversations life throws at you with poise and assurance. Investing in yourself through education, skills development, and furthering your career are key elements to obtaining such confidence. The world is ever evolving, and one must stay abreast of the latest developments and innovations to strive for excellence in their field while making sure to always keep their confidence at the helm. Going beyond one's comfort zone and taking on projects that push your boundaries are essential skills for a powerful man and can only be obtained by a strong sense of self-assurance.

YOU ARE SIGNIFICANT

"Men are important and valued. Keep fighting and don't give up".

"Men have played an important role on the earth since time existed. They have been the protectors, providers, and leaders for their families, communities, and civilizations. Their existence holds great importance in maintaining order, progress, and stability in society".

As fathers, men provide guidance, care, and discipline to their children which helps shape future generations. They teach their sons the virtues of hard work, perseverance, integrity, and responsible living. They mold their daughters into caring, empathetic, and ambitious women.

As leaders in business, politics, religion, and other fields, men have established rules, institutions, and infrastructure that have helped advance human progress. From inventing tools and machines to establishing legal and political systems, men have contributed greatly to building modern civilization.

Even in moments of crisis and conflict, men have stepped up as warriors and defenders to save lives and protect communities. Their courage and sacrifice have safeguarded culture, religion, and values that uphold the moral fabric of society.

While women play an equally important role in nurturing life and maintaining harmony, men, and women complement each other and together create a balanced world. The existence of both genders is essential for a healthy and prosperous society.

Men throughout history have forged the world we live in today through their ideas, inventions, and achievements. They have pushed the boundaries of what was thought possible and advanced human civilization.

Some of the greatest men in history include:

Martin Luther King Jr. was an iconic leader in the American civil rights movement from the 1950s until his assassination in 1968. King sought equality and human rights for African Americans, the poor, and all victims of injustice through peaceful protest.

Barack Obama served as the 44th president of the United States from 2009 to 2017. He was the first African American president in the country's history. Before becoming president, Obama represented Illinois in the United States Senate from 2005 to 2008.

Albert Einstein developed the theories of relativity and changed our understanding of space, time, matter, and the universe.

Frederick Douglass was an African American social reformer, abolitionist, orator, writer, and statesman. After escaping from slavery, he became a leader of the abolitionist movement, gaining note for his dazzling oratory and incisive antislavery writing.

Thomas Edison invented the light bulb and phonograph, transforming how we light our world and listen to music.

Benjamin Banneker was an African American scientist, surveyor, almanac author, and farmer. He is known for his survey of the initial boundaries of the District of Columbia. Banneker also published an almanac yearly from 1792 to 1797.

Wright brothers who achieved the first powered flight and paved the way for air travel and aviation.

Great men have improved our lives in countless ways. However, not all geniuses get the chance to change the world. Many great minds are lost due to persecution, oppression, violence, and conflict.

It is important that we protect and nurture the gifted among us to allow their talents to flourish. We must build a society that allows great men to achieve their full potential for the benefit of humanity.

Safeguarding great minds and allowing them to do their life's work means ensuring equity, justice, peace, and the freedoms that enable them to create and innovate. This will help ensure the progress of civilization and secure a better future for our children.

DISCLAIMER

This information is for informational purposes only and is not intended to treat, diagnose, or cure any illnesses or diseases. Please consult a qualified healthcare professional for personalized medical advice.

C. Anglin

www.ingramcontent.com/pod-product-compliance
Lightning Source LLC
Chambersburg PA
CBHW050047260726
48658CB00005B/1820